KRATOM

KRATOM FOR BEGINNERS,

EVERYTHING YOU NEED TO KNOW ABOUT KRATOM

DR. Christopher Nash

Kratom

Copyright 2016 - All Rights Reserved

ALL RIGHTS RESERVED. No part of this publication may be reproduced or transmitted in any form whatsoever, electronic, or mechanical, including photocopying, recording, or by any informational storage or retrieval system without express written, dated and signed permission from the author.

Table of Contents

INTRODUCTION 4
OVERVIEW 6
BRIEF HISTORY OF KRATOM..11
LEVELS OF EFFECT 17
KRATOM DOSAGE AND ITS EFFECTS..22
KRATOM'S LEGAL STATUS 31
Q AND A..38
THE ADVOCACY IN FAVOUR OF KRATOM 42
HOW KRATOM IS PRODUCED AND IT'S USES?...........................46
KRATOM EXTRACT GUIDE 53
PREPARATION AND CONSUMPTION 57
CONTROVERSIES AROUND KRATOM 66
CONCLUSION..68

INTRODUCTION

We are all aware of the beneficial qualities of almost all kinds and 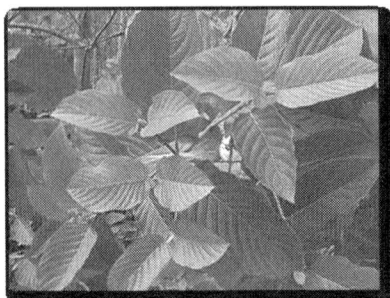 varieties of coffee. We are also very much aware of the side-effects if we consume too much of it.

As the ancient Greeks maintained, every moderation is perfection, so no compound, regardless of how beneficial it might be, should be consumed uncontrollably. This is the case with a variety of coffee indigenous to Southeast Asia (Indochina, Malaysia and Thailand, which is becoming rapidly known under the names of kratum, ketum or, as most people know it, kratom.

There has been a lot of controversy in reference to its effects on humans and on occasion its use, possession and purchase have been either completely prohibited by law, or it has been deemed as a controlled substance with adverse effects if consumed in greater quantities than the safety limit set.

This controversy is the result of insufficient scientific research conducted on the subject which would resolve the issue and set the record straight on what is and what is not safe. As we will see this research has met with various kinds of difficulties and obstacles that are not directly linked with Kratom itself.

The people in Southeast Asia have been using it for a long time before it was discovered and classified by Dutch botanist Pieter korthals. The relevant joke on the discovery is that Korthals gave it the scientific name Mitragyna because the shape of the leaf stripes reminded him of a bishop's miter!

As we will discuss further in the following chapters, Kratom has a lot of medicinal and recreational uses. The people of Thailand, where the greatest concentrations of the plant are observed, consume as much as 70 leaves per day just by chewing them.

For them it can be used as a traditional form of medicine to fight pain, as an antidiarrheal, to treat people that are dependent upon the use of opioids, even as a remedy for premature ejaculation during sexual intercourse. Many of them begin using it at the age of 25 and continue to do so for the rest of their lives. Usually they start with 10 leaves per day and gradually increase the intake to 60 or 70.

The first real indication of the wisdom involved is that even the Thais do not start using it before they are 25 which makes it question worthy why the western medicine does not take this fact into account.

It should be made perfectly clear at this point and before we go any further, that it is not the intention of this book to present a case that contradicts the applicable laws in the various jurisdictions. The contents are purely informative and under no circumstances it can be considered that they are intended to provide a basis for usage against legal provisions. If the law in your jurisdiction forbids its use, please do not use it.

Let's begin unraveling the mysteries, the misunderstandings, the misconceptions and the facts that surround this plant.

OVERVIEW

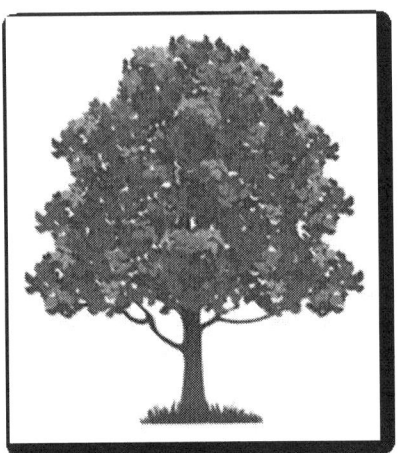

Kratom is a tree that reaches an average of 30 feet high and 15 feet wide. There have been cases of 70 feet high trees but those are rather rare. Depending on the climate it is cultivated and the environment it can have a color that varies from evergreen to deciduous. The leaves are about 7 inches long and 4 inches wide and the flowers are round and yellow growing in clusters at the end of the tree branches.

The usable part by humans are the leaves. The can be consumed raw (chewed), dried, in powder mixed with water, or in the form of a boiled tea. The common people of Southeast Asia prefer chewing it and have been using it for basically two reasons: to lift their moods and as a stimulant, much in the same way as westerners drink coffee or tea. It helped them a lot to carry out their very long and monotonous daily work duties.

However, those with a greater understanding of the plant attribute management of chronic pain to its qualities along with the capability to be used as an opium substitute and an opium dependency management drug, an antidiarrheal and as a remedy to premature ejaculation during sexual intercourse. Occasional but not excessive use provides enough energy boost and levels of relaxation to maintain the body in balance.

Initial research showed more than 40 chemicals that gave Kratom its qualities. Among these chemicals are alkaloids like mitragynine and mitraphylline, raubasine and corynantheidine. Originally it was thought that mitragynine was the basic active ingredient until it was discovered that the content of 7-hydroxymitragynine is what gives Kratom its chemical properties.

It is classified as a psychoactive compound acting much like morphine but without the hypoventilation that is typical of the use of morphine and with completely dissimilar effects which are attributed to the mix of alkaloids which seem to have both stimulating and sedative effects.

In low to moderate doses, Kratom is definitely a stimulant causing a heightened state of alertness in the mind, more physical energy and the ability to get through a day of monotonous work. Furthermore, it loosens the tongues (i.e. people are more talkative), and makes people friendlier and more sociable.

A higher dose will definitely have a sedative effect. This dosage is used to fight chronic pain, the effects of opiate withdrawal and symptoms of anxiety. It may be possible that there will be some nausea present which will dissipate quickly upon lying down and relaxing.

The tricky part is the moderate dosage. After a certain level and before it becomes a sedative, Kratom has the ability to provide the much prized state of being between waking and dreaming. Officially this is called the euphoric-analgesic state and it is the state that most romantic writers of the 19th century resorted to narcotics and opium derivatives to achieve.

The danger involved in the consumption of Kratom comes from the different varieties. The usual leaves that are consumed raw by chewing very rarely have presented adverse side-effects as long as their use is occasional and not uncontrollable.

However, in the powdered form that is used to produce tea or even worse in its extract forms which are much more potent, it is possible to develop dependencies much like the consumption of tobacco and alcohol and to present side-effects in the form of nausea, bowel obstruction, runny nose, and irritability, loss of weight and appetite and diarrhea. Fortunately, all these side-effects retreat quickly and are easily treatable.

Two things are absolutely forbidden when it comes to consumption of Kratom. The first one is to drive. It has been documented that the stimulating effect of Kratom makes drivers more prone to road rage, while the sedative and euphoric effects tend to distract the attention from the road and lead directly to accidents.

The second one is that under no circumstances it is to be used by women during their pregnancy. There has been absolutely no research conducted as to the effects it may have on the fetus. Until it is scientifically proven that no deformities or other problems befall upon the children it is strongly recommended to err on the side of caution.

Some heated debate has been raised as to the effect that Kratom has when it is mixed with other drugs. Even though it is well-known that mixing drugs is a problem, there are those who maintain that it is not Kratom that is at fault in such a case. There have been three documented cases of deaths on this (mixture with the drug tramadol); therefore, it is strongly recommended not to mix Kratom with any other forms of prescription medication without receiving proper advice and guidance by a proper medical professional. For obvious reasons it is suggested that this professional should be relatively open minded.

Mixture with other kinds of tea has not presented any problems even though officially kratom is a variety of coffee. In fact there are recipes that mix kratom with green or black tea. The same stand true with other herbs. However, it should be made sure first that the contents of the mixture in chemicals do not contradict or react with each other to create a medical problem.

In the next chapter we will discuss the effect levels of each different variety to see how much of it has been documented as safe for use.

Kratom

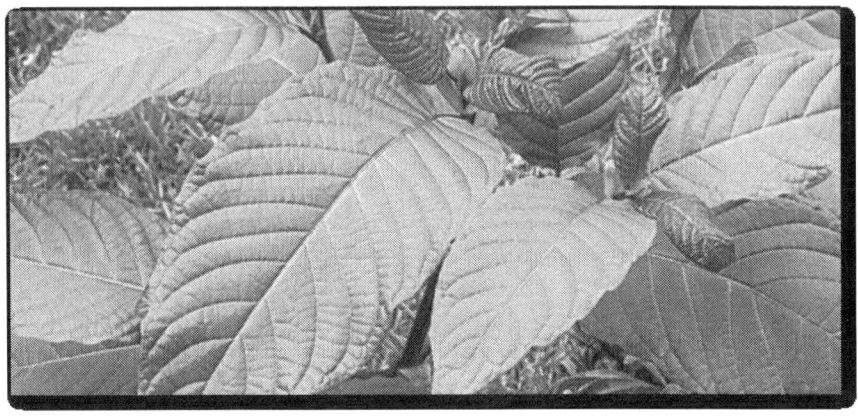

BRIEF HISTORY OF KRATOM

In the year 1930 in Thailand, the very first regulation of opium was proclaimed. This granted the authority and power to officers to capture dependents of the drug and traffickers till they combat the addiction. It was in the year 1913 when the Cocaine and Morphine Act B.E. 2456 conquers the importation of cocaine and morphine in the kingdom.

In the year 1922, Narcotics Act B.E. 2465 was founded as a result of the International Opium Convention which was attended by Thailand in the year 1914 in Hague, Netherlands. This law regulates all the action for drugs like sale, consumption, possession, production and importation.

In the year 1934, the Cannabis Act was pronounced to safeguard the citizen from cannabis addiction. It was in the year 1939 when the Kratom Act was declared to regulate the proliferation and harvest of Kratom trees. Moreover, there are several laws in Thailand that have something to do with drugs where kratom falls in the mentioned category. Essentially, this is primarily because of the effects of drug which Kratom can provide.

Kratom Defined

Mitragyna Speciosa or simply Kratom is known as a native tree that can usually be found in Borneo, Indonesia, Malaysia, Thailand and other Southeast Asian countries. Other names used for Kratom include Ketum, Thom, Ithang and Kakuam. It comes from the family of Rubiaceae where coffee tree also comes from. This herbal drug's leaves have been utilized as a useful herbal medication in lineage medicine particularly as a pain killer, stimulant at low dosages, drug treatment for diarrhea, recreational drug, an effective treatment for opiate addiction and sedative at high dosages.

Kratom is viewed as one of the most pleasurable and potent psychoactive herbs that is ready for use nowadays. This herb's effects usually last for about four up to six hours. Some residual effects may remain for fewer hours longer when huge amount of kratom is consumed. On the other hand, fatigue may be reduced and the user may experience mild euphoria when low dosage is consumed. Low dosages do not meddle with ordinary activities, but, the user should not do other activities which need concentration such as driving. Take note that when kratom is taken in high dosage, its effects are strongly pleasurable and gives you a feeling of being so enchanted.

Generally, users describe the effects as ecstatic, heavenly and elated. A lot of people experience visuals which are described as closed-eye. High dosage must only be consumed when a person can commit more time to experience itself.

Scientific Studies of Kratom

A considerable number of people are curious about Kratom leaves. As a matter of fact, certain firms such as pharmaceutical and scientific groups are facilitating research regarding the properties, composition and effects of this herb in people. Kratom is broadly available at present in the market due to its easy access online. Studies revealed that the herb is being abused mainly because of the effects that it can provide to the people who consume it. In Southeast Asia, Japan and USA, certain clinical researches are being administered to further test the leaves of kratom.

Up until today, the effects of this herb are not yet completely understood. Current research just disclosed that the herb's leaves contain alkaloids which can affect the brain's mu-opioid receptor. In addition to this, alkaloids such as mitragyne can provide specific effects like depressing and stimulating traits. Meanwhile, the process with regards to how these alkaloids function and affect a person's behavior is yet to uncover.

Furthermore, it has been shown that kratom can be an effective pain reliever even though there are actually no commercially ready for use pills or preparations which are made from the leaves of this herb. It has also been found that this herb can aid r educe withdrawal symptoms of those individuals who are already dependent on morphine and opiate. In rehabilitation therapy, this herb serves as a great alternative to opiates and it is known to provide subtler withdrawal symptoms as compared to those of opiates. Due to this, scientists perceive kratom as a future substance which can be used as a drug to defeat dependence and drug addiction.

What is more, it has been unveiled that this herb is an efficient stimulant. In connection to this, future efforts are being made in order to come up with effective and strong kratom-based antidepressants. However, this plan will surely go a long way since it is necessary to acquire more exhaustive research and deeper understanding of the behavioral activities as well as moods of the brain and its receptors.

In actuality, there are also some efforts in formulating cosmetics which are kratom-based. Besides the reality that this herb can have impact on a person's mind, research reveals that this herb leaf can also affect the body once it is topically applied to the skin. Future skin lotions and rejuvenating creams which are kratom-based are also being studied and are some things to look forward to in the future.

How is kratom taken?

Hinging on a person's preference, this drug can be consumed by several approaches. The leaves of Kratom are commonly chewed fresh (typically after taking off the fibrous main vein) in Thailand. Also, dried kratom leaves can be chewed as well; however, since these are slightly tough, a great number of individual choose to crush them or take them in powder form so it can be easily swallowed. The powder form can be combined with water. This approach is fast and easy. Further, it is slightly bitter-tasting when swallowed and a bit fibrous smoothie. You may consider combining it with apple sauce or fruit juice. The dried leaves of kratom are typically made into a tea which is first strained and then drunk.

It is essential to note that tea is a lot easier to drink as compared to powdered Kratom that is suspended in water. This can be smoked; however, it may be impractical since the amount of leaf which makes up a common dose is too much to be easily smoked. More than that, a paste-like extract can be prepared through evaporating the water from the kratom tea. This may be set aside for later use. Small shots of this extract may be swallowed or you may prefer dissolving it in hot water and be taken as a tea. There are some people who prefer to combine ordinary black tea with kratom tea or other herbal teas prior it is consumed. In so doing, it tastes better. If you prefer to sweeten it, honey or sugar may be added.

Procedure in Making Kratom Tea

The procedure below is a fundamental recipe for making kratom tea. This makes adequate tea for a few doses-approximately eight slightly strong doses, if using high quality kratom:

a) Take about 56 grams or 2 ounces of crushed or dried kratom leaves and afterwards place this into a pot. Then, you may add roughly 1 liter of 1 quart of water.

b) For 15 minutes, allow it to boil.

c) Then, it is time to pour the tea using a strainer into the bowl and then reserve the liquid. Take note that you have to thoroughly squeeze the leaves in the strainer so you can get the most of the liquid out.

d) Gently put the kratom leaves back in the pot and then add another liter of fresh water. Then, do steps 2 and 3 again. But, this time, after the leaves have been thoroughly strained for the second time, they can be disposed.

e) Finally, you have to put the mixed liquid from both boilings back into the pot. After that, it is time to boil it till the volume is reduced to approximately 250 ml or one cup.

Be reminded that the purpose here is to boil the tea down to a low volume in order for each single dose to be immediately swallowed. This can be boiled down to any concentration you prefer. Be extra cautious at the near end of the procedure because once this begins to become syrupy, it may burn or spatter.

Due to the fact that the tea comes with a bitter taste, you may consider gulping it down fast and then chase it with a few good-tasting fruit juice at once to reduce the not-so-good taste.

Moreover, the same universal preparation approach can be utilized with smaller or bigger amounts of herb through merely adjusting the volume of the water utilized. You can safely set aside the kratom tea in the fridge for approximately 5 days. It is perhaps all right to keep it a bit longer; however, it is much better to be extra careful and no longer drink it after 5 days. If you add some alcohol to it, it is possible for the tea to be stored in several months.

By adding roughly 10% of alcohol, the tea may be stored for several months in the fridge. Some ingredients may precipitate out of solution especially when placed in the fridge and this creates sediment in the container's bottom. The sediment may contain alkaloids so this means that it is crucial to re-dissolve it prior drinking the tea. Through stirring and warming the tea, this can be easily re-dissolved.

LEVELS OF EFFECT

Kratom is categorized in five levels of effect that depend upon the potency of the variety used. The classification is highly dependent upon the sensitivity of each individual; therefore, it should be considered that each level of effect is not an exact match but a rather loose affiliation. They also depend greatly upon whether the user takes kratom on an empty stomach, or if the use occurs after a meal.

These five levels are:

A) **The threshold**
In this level the stimulating and mood enhancing effects are subtle but clearly apparent. This usually occurs at very low to low doses of up to medium potency of kratom.

B) **Mild**
The stimulation is clearly apparent and well felt. So is the mood uplifting. Depending on the potency and the tolerance developed by the body it occurs at low doses of medium potency or moderate doses of standard potency.

C) **Moderate**
This is the level that balances between stimulation and the sedative-euphoric-analgesic effects. It can occur at a number of combinations of dosage and potency and is subject greatly upon the tolerance and the sensitivity level of each individual.

D) **Strong**

Highly sensitive people find this level too strong and cannot support it. For the others it's the level where the effects have become clearly sedative and border to the euphoric and analgesic ones. It is the level required for those suffering from high anxiety issues and need to relax and for those who need to get some sleep and do not want to use synthetic sleeping pills.

E) **Very strong**
For most people this is a level that they cannot stand. It's a very strongly sedative level where the euphoric effects border with hallucination. Usually it occurs after an immensely great quantity of kratom has been consumed of either low or medium potency or the maximum safe dosage of a kratom extract has been exceeded.

To understand the correlation between the potency and the levels of effect, every leaf that is consumed raw counts for 2 grams of low potency. The following chart shows the dosages that have been tested for safety:

Level	Low potency	Medium Potency	Extracts
Threshold	2-4 grams	1-3 grams	1 gram
Mild	3-5 grams	2-4 grams	1-2 grams
Moderate	4-10 grams	3-7 grams	2-4 grams
Strong	8-15 grams	6-10 grams	3-6 grams
Very strong	12-25 grams	8-16 grams	5-8 grams

It is clearly evident that the extracts are much more potent than the rest of the forms of kratom and extreme care should be given to their consumption. Extracts are the main ingredient of the kratom capsules that have been circulated on the market and the absence of the correct warnings is one of the factors that have led to the current disinformation that exists.

There are six major varieties of kratom. The following image displays their potencies in reference to the energy boost, the relaxation effect and the mood enhancing properties of each. The properties are attributed to the raw leaves which always hold the lowest value as far as potency is concerned. The leaf color depicted is also an indication of the correct tint to expect for the premium quality of each variety.

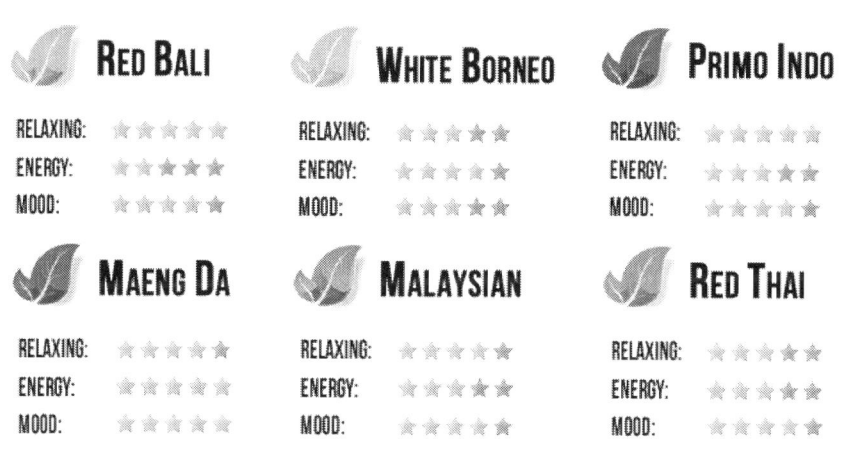

At any potency or level of effect, kratom lasts for 5 or 6 hours. If it's taken on an empty stomach the effects are evident after 30 to 40 minutes. After a meal it will take between 60 and 90 minutes to feel the effects. It takes even longer if it is consumed in the form of capsules where it will take some time for the outside shell to dissolve and the best time to use kratom is three hours after a meal.

Further to the warnings about driving and women in pregnancy it is recommended not to climb ladders or use any power tools after having taken kratom. It is also advisable not to leave a pot on a stove and go to sleep (that's valid for anything actually).

Talking about the effects and the potencies does not give you an idea on how to consume it. The people where the tree grows up indigenously just chew the leaves. This is rather difficult for westerners. In the next chapter we will discuss how to prepare and consume kratom.

The Adverse Effects of Taking Kratom

This herbal drug is a distinctive drug because a mild to average dosage will commonly be stimulating. Meanwhile, high dosage is nearly often very sedating. This is due to the fact that the active alkaloids contain sedative and stimulant effects. Indeed, which dominates perhaps hinges on both the individual and dosage variances between users. There are a lot of reports that the effects are very identical to those of opiate drugs. This is no longer surprising from a pharmacological point of view since kratom actually have alkaloids which act as opiate receptor agonists. Kratom does not seem to be quite addictive even though it comes with identical mechanism of action as several opiate pain medications. As a matter of fact, a lot of people utilize kratom to get over opiate addiction.

- **The stimulant level**

At this phase, sexual and physical energy is increased, the brain becomes more active, a person becomes more sociable, friendly and talkative and, capable of doing very tedious physical work. There are a number of people who find this phase jittery rather than good.

- **The sedative-ecstatic-soother level**

At this phase, a person will look and feel calm, be less delicate to emotional as well as physical pain, may experience a good dreamy reverie, have a feeling of pleasure and comfort. However, a person may also feel nauseous but this may ease off once you relax, feel some sweating or itching and suffer from constricted pupils. Likewise, you may notice that your appreciation to music is highly enhanced.

You will have the feeling that it is absolutely very pleasurable to relax while eyes are closed and being in a relaxing and semi-darkened spot listening to your most preferred music. This experience also makes the person delight in the opportunity to feel like dreaming and waking at the same time. It is like being both in the real world and in the fantasy world. Romantic writers in the nineteenth century desired for this form of state and most of them resorted to opium (which is perceived as a habit-forming drug to obtain a combined state of dreaming and waking) since they weren't still aware of kratom.

KRATOM DOSAGE AND ITS EFFECTS

Warning:

People do differ when it comes to susceptibility to kratom. In the same way, kratom from various sources can also differ in terms of potency. This makes it especially vital for dosage estimates to be considered as loose estimates. A person must always begin with a mild dosage particularly when he or she is still sampling with a new set of kratom.

A person may then maximize the dosage gradually with succeeding experiments till he or she acquires the preferred effects level. For first timers, it is not advised to take a more dosage when you are still experimenting on a new set of this herbal leaf. Countless of people suffer from nausea when using very strong dosage. On the other hand, sensitive people may encounter sickness even with milder dosages. Some individuals are hypersensitive to kratom and due to this they may encounter adverse reactions when using very strong dosages like prolonged and severe vomiting.

Why is it essential to start by determining the right dose?

Prior starting to experiment with methods on how to consume or take kratom, it is deemed necessary to compute the right dosage for you. Apart from which strain you prefer, the dosage is considered as one of the most valuable part of utilizing this drug as an herbal medicinal.

Take into account that numbers can actually differ broadly hinged on the potency of the powder you select, whether or not there is added extract or whether you prefer a more relaxing and energizing experience. Always remember that personal tolerance is also vital here just like how rested the user is, the general body type as well as your emotional frame of mind.

It matters to think of all these vital factors when computing a dosage. Indeed, it may take a lot of sessions over weeks or months prior a person obtain his or her precise kratom dose determined; however, this is all right. What matters most is that you are respectful of the procedure. The amount of threshold for nearly all strains is one gram. Take note that this is often a great beginning point.

It is wise to remember that smaller dosages absolutely produce more invigorating effects while higher dosages are perceived to have more of a calming property.

Why Use Kratom?

This drug has been utilized for centuries in Southeast Asian countries mainly because it has been proven to have effective pain-killing properties even though neither its alkaloids nor the drug itself has been used in contemporary medicine. As compared to morphine, mitragynine contains less pain-killing effects; however, it does not cause considerable dependence, thus, making it feasibly beneficial in treating mild to moderate sorts of discomfort or pain.

Universally, there is a great amount of mitragynine contained in the plant of a kratom, this actually makes it efficient to extract for use when it comes to managing pain. In relation to this, the 7-hydrohydroxymitragynine has been revealed to contain more vigorous pain-killing effects; however, it is less ample as compared to mitragynine which is contained in the Kratom plant.

Indeed, it may not be useful to extract these alkaloids from the plant of kratom utilizing the modern technology; however, if mitragynine can be transformed into 7-hydrohydroxymitragynine, then, this may eventually emerge as an all-natural as well as a less expensive replacement for contemporary medications for pain management.

The Duration of Effects when taking Kratom

Typically, the effects of kratom last for five up to six hours. The onset of effects is commonly felt thirty by up to forty minutes after ingestion when this drug is taken when a person did not consume any food. Meanwhile, when the person is full or have much food in his or her stomach, it may take approximately an hour and a half prior it starts to take effect. The onset of effects may be put off slightly when taken in vegetarian or gelatin capsules since it takes time for these capsules to dissolve.

What is the duration of kratoms effects?

The effects of kratom usually last 5-6 hours. When taken on an empty stomach, the onset of effects is typically felt 30-40 minutes after ingestion. If there is much food in the stomach, it may take 60-90 minutes before it begins to take effect. When taken in capsules (gelatin or vegetarian), the onset of effects may be delayed a little because it takes time for the capsules to dissolve in the stomach.

How safe is Kratom and what are the risks you must expect when taking it?

When taking kratom without combining it with other medications or narcotics, a person using it may feel sleepy while doing risky activities. For this reason, it is advised not to drive, climb ladders or utilize power tools when this herbal drug is taken even though you feel perked up. Drowsiness may come without caution. Always be wary and do not do things which you are potentially hazardous and then fall asleep.

Women who are preginate are not advised to take any medication or narcotic except of course when prescribed by a doctor. Due to the fact that there've been no researches regarding the perils of kratom intake by expecting women, it is not clearly known if this could really cause fetal death or birth defects. This is the main reason why it is strongly advised that pregnant women not use this herbal drug.

Counterfeit Kratom

Counterfeit Kratom has also been widely sold. This fabricated Kratom has been sold by a few vendors using the name of mellow gold. In line with this, there have been several reports of counterfeit Kratom being sold before; however, this seems that most Kratom available on the market these days are now genuine. In truth, it is not known what plant or herb matter was certainly being sold as kratom; however, it is speculated that it is from a type of tree in the same genus family.

It is important to know that kratom was uncovered to be adulterer with a synthetic opiate known as the O-desmethyl-tramadol. Many overdoses have taken place between the year 2009 and 2011 and some of these even resulted to several cases of fatalities.

Kratom Pies

There are some vendors who currently began selling kratom pies. These appear to be the newest version of extracts mainly because the original ones did not work out well. The reason behind this is because a lot of consumers were not delighted with them.

Even though these are rather high-priced, a lot of consumers have positive experiences with the products. As a matter of fact, they have been regarded as quite easy to handle. Aside from this, the vendors sell the extract of kratom in pies and assert that you could create tiny spills out of them and then you just have to swallow them. Please be guided that this is not true as this will not dissolve easily in the stomach.

The Dangers of Kratom

In the past, kratom was used by the natives as medicine for some sorts of pain and discomfort and also for diarrhea. Aside from this, people who are addicted or dependent on morphine and opiates are encountering withdrawal symptoms when they cease consuming the narcotic. Medicinal method was substantiated to utilize kratom as a substitute to morphine and opium. It was confirmed that giving this drug in low dosage then slowly reduced until total withdrawal leads to safer and milder withdrawal symptoms as compared to opiates and morphine withdrawal symptoms. More than that, there are other perks that kratom reports to provide.

Is kratom considered a very efficient medication for discomfort or other forms of pain?

A great number of people claim that kratom is a very efficient soother or pain medication. As a matter of fact, it is regarded as the most efficient herbal pain medication available these days aside from opium.

Is kratom regarded as a very efficient treatment for opiate addiction?

In truth, one of the conventional uses of this herbal drug in Thailand is as an efficient treatment for people who are suffering from opiate addiction which is known as a globally widespread issue these days. This is beneficial not only to people who utilize opiate drugs illegally, it is also helpful for those who are prescribed with opiate pain narcotics. Sadly, those who use opiate medications every day usually become addicted to it.

Naturally, a lot of people do not prefer being addicted to these medications and are definitely searching for ways to overpower their addiction. Over and above, plenty of people claim that kratom is quite efficient when it comes to this purpose. Since kratom has alkaloids which certainly function as opiate receptor agonists, this herbal drug can be utilized as an alternative for opiate medications, both as to effectively avoid opiate withdrawals and as an effective medication to pain or any discomfort. This clearly means that kratom varies from opiate drugs in a very valuable and useful manner. So, prior deciding to use kratom to defeat opiate addiction, it is of course quite imperative to consult a physician first.

Is kratom drug habit forming?

This herbal drug is actually not habit forming especially when it is used with a purpose, in other words, it is more beneficial when used responsibly. The good news is that there is no danger of becoming overly dependent to kratom when it is used infrequently rather than on a daily basis. However, it is deemed essential not to get into the habit of using this herbal drug daily. The reason behind this is because kratom just like other forms of drugs could become a habit that is difficult to break specifically when used for a prolonged period or taken every day.

Be reminded that prior beginning the experiment, it is wise to set some usage guidelines. Take into account that if you ever find it so complicated to stay within the usage guidelines set, then, it is better to stop using this herbal drug. However, individuals who use kratom on the purpose of beating a foregoing opiate addiction may be required to use kratom on a daily basis in order for him or her to inhibit opiate withdrawal.

In line with this, individuals who experience chronic pain may necessarily take medications to manage pain every day. Some individuals prefer to use kratom rather than other pharmaceutical pain relievers. It is interesting to note that some researches have revealed that opiate medications like morphine are barely addictive for people who suffer from pain expect among those with a history of drug abuse. This is perhaps also true for kratom since just like opiate drugs, its effects are mainly due to the activity of opiate receptor agonist.

The Risk-free Usage Guidelines

As always, it is best to be cautious especially because it concerns one's health. For that reason, it is recommended that people not use kratom more than once per week. It is advised to take kratom at least once or twice per month. In so doing, you will be assured that this herbal drug will not become a habit that is difficult to break. It should be considered as an occasional treat and not as something that is taken on a daily basis to prevent addiction and other adverse effects. This way, there is no reason for an individual to worry about habituation and at the same time obtain more pleasure from using this herbal drug.

Are there any claimed or recorded health issues?

Health issues are not probable unless a person is using or taking huge dosage of kratom on a regular basis. It has been reported that some individuals in Thailand who consume kratom daily and who are already dependent on it suffer from physical withdrawal symptoms especially when they suddenly stop, dark pigmentation in the face area and noticeable weight loss.

Some people claim that this herb enables them to perform sexually with more vigor, excitement and for longer period of time than the usual. To some, kratom minimizes the sensitivity to sexual organs, in this manner; it takes more time to reach an orgasm. This drug appears to have a not so good effect on the user's sexual performance though and many users claim to experience brief erectile problems.

Further, withdrawal symptoms comprise of crying, muscle jerking, muscle aches, runny nose, diarrhea and irritability. Health issues are rare to take place in kratom users who consume the herbal drug occasionally. Just like any medicine or drug, the reactions of people differ even though kratom is used responsibly.

The human body may actually develop tolerance against the alkaloids which are contained in mitragyna. This may create the need to maximize the dosage to obtain the preferred effects. When kratom is consumed in higher dosage (overdose), the person may experience, restlessness, delusion, hallucinations, tremors, nausea as well as coordination problems.

Due to this, daily consumption of this drug for a long time is not advised as this may lead to nervousness, skin darkening, constipation and aggression. If you are suffering from ulcers, schizophrenia, hepatic problems, renal and cardiac issues and low blood pressure, this drug is not recommended for you to use.

Is it possible to combine kratom safely with other drugs?

Needless to say, combining substances can generally be dangerous. So, it is advisable not to combine kratom with huge dosage of caffeine, yohimbine, amphetamine-like substances and cocaine as these drugs when combined with kratom can potentially increase a person's blood pressure and he or she may be overly stimulated. Likewise, do not mix kratom with opiates, huge amount of alcohol as well as benzodiazepines or any substances which are known to have the capability to weaken the body's immune system. It is important to understand that these combinations may lead to over-sedation and the person may also suffer from difficulty in breathing. This can be lethal and serious particularly if MAO inhibitor substances are mixed with monoamine drugs. Meanwhile, the combination of kratom and MAO inhibitor substances has not yet been exhaustively researched.

Additionally, some combinations have been claimed by users to be supposedly risk-free and quite pleasant. Kratom can be mixed with an ordinary tea safely. In point of fact, kratom has been used with a tea that is especially made from Papaver rhoeas or simply known as red poppy flowers. This comes with a sedating-ecstatic tea that is made from Nymphaea caerulea (blue lotus) and also comes with intensely low narcotic effect.

Indeed, kratom has been mixed safely with low quantities of alcohol; be that as it may, huge quantities of alcohol should be refrained from. There are some people who claim that they prefer to smoke cannabis or tobacco while using kratom. However, it is crucial for someone smoking while using kratom to be extra careful not to drop lit smoking items or take a nap during the activity.

KRATOM'S LEGAL STATUS

The Legal Status of Kratom

Kratom was utilized as a medicinal herb to treat some ailments such as diarrhea and pain by ancient cultures. In truth, this herb's functions effects and compositions are not yet entirely understood. The kratom tree is quite large in number in Thailand. The good thing about this herb is that they do not have to be cultivated since they are easy to access. The herb's leaves can be boiled, smoked or chewed and also utilized as tea by countless of natives. Age-old Asian cultures utilized this herb for such a long time for nearly more than centuries now.

Additionally, the chemical components of kratom disclose that the herb's leaves have alkaloids like mitragyne which has noticeable effects to the brain's mu-opioid receptors. As revealed by some researches, this herb comes with intoxicating, stimulating and depressing effects. Even though the precise functions on how the alkaloids of this herb really works and how they affect the brain is not completely understood, still, a lot of scientists perceive that this herb can be utilized as a drug or medicinal substance. People suffering from morphine and opiate addiction and dependence are experiencing withdrawal symptoms when there is sudden cessation of the consumption of the said narcotic.

Studies uncovered that kratom can be utilized as a great alternative to morphine and opiates in order to reduce the dangers of withdrawal symptoms. This herb can certainly provide safer and lesser withdrawal symptoms as compared to morphine and opiates. This drug is given in a low and regulated dosage and then the dosage is reduced until the total withdrawal. While there are no records or claims of the negative effects of kratom, if this herb is given and consumed in higher dose, consumed on a daily basis or more regularly for a long period of time, then, this may also come with adverse effects such as addiction, hence, making this herb another substance to be abused. Because of this, the legalities of this herb are being questioned by different countries' governments.

More than that, independent researches about this herb are being administered for the purpose of setting grounds in prohibiting or controlling the use of the drug. Various nations have different laws against narcotics. In Canada and other countries, kratom is not yet fully regulated. In Thailand which is known as the herb's native land, mitragyna is actually not allowed. Also, possessing specific dosage or amount of this herb is punishable by their laws.

This herbal drug is also prohibited in Myanmar, Australia, Thailand, Malaysia and Denmark. Some of these countries establish very severe dues or punishment for the possession and use of this herbal drug. However, this herb is legal in some countries such as in most part of Europe and in USA. So, it is critical to learn if kratom is legal in your country first prior to using this herb. Take note that laws and regulations in your country can and do change.

This herb is regarded as not prohibited in most states in USA but not in Vermont and Indiana. Kratom is also legal in some parts of Europe. This simply conveys that all parts of this herb as well as it extracts are legit to purchase, grow, possess, give, trade, sell or distribute without the need for prescription or license. If this drug is sold as a supplement, take into account that the sales should adhere to the supplement laws of US. On the other hand, if it is sold for consumptions as drug or food, then, sales must be administered by the FDA.

Kratom

List of countries where kratom is illegal:

- Romania
- Bulgaria
- Finland
- South Korea
- Poland
- Sweden
- Israel
- Denmark
- Thailand
- Lithuania
- New Zealand
- Malaysia
- Norway
- Burma (Myanmar)
- Ireland
- Australia

Kratom

In some parts of USA, here are the regions where kratom is not allowed:

- Illinois
- Tennessee
- Louisiana
- Wisconsin
- Indiana

In the United Kingdom, kratom can be bought without a prescription. In addition to this, it is not recently restricted or scheduled. Ina actuality, there are some local vendors of kratom capsules and powder in UK; however, they are a lot more high-priced as compared to retailers who are based in North America.

On the other hand, in Canada, kratom is allowed. It can actually be used, sold and bought without any restrictions.

Whether or not this herb is beneficial or addictive just like other substances out there, it is always best to be very careful, responsible and disciplined. There is nothing wrong if the herb is used for medicinal and other good purposes and if it is consumed in right amount. What makes it wrong is when the drug is abused and used for negative purposes. Nowadays, in spite of harsh words and issues on illegalities of kratom in some countries, regions and in some parts of Thailand, peasants as well as natives carry on using this herb. In reality, attempts to shatter wild kratom trees have had insignificant effect since the tree is known as a native to Thailand. At present, this drug ranks as top 2 in prohibited drugs in Thailand. What is more, there are hearsays that Thailand may phase out the hugely unsuccessful ban of the controversial tree.

The Active Components of Kratom

This herb contains over twenty-five alkaloids. Aside from the two primary alkaloids mentioned above, other alkaloids present in kratom include oxindoles, speciofoline, paynanthine, mitraphylline, speciogynine, ajmalicine, mitraversine, stipulatine, corynanthedine and the rhychophylline.

In reality, there are several closely-linked tryptamine alkaloids found in kratom. And, the most valuable ones are 7-hydroxymitragynine and mitragynine. To boot, these are mainly responsible for the herbal drug's sedative, stimulating, pain relieving and euphoric effects. Tryptamine alkaloids actually look like yohimbine in terms of structure; however, these do not have similar effects.

Is Kratom Use Possibly Detected on Drug Examinations?

Even though kratom does not have alkaloids which relate to opiate receptors, these are basically unrelated to opiate substances and hence would not be spotted through opiate drug examinations. On the other hand, it is technically probable to uncover the alkaloids contained in kratom in body fluids; however, because kratom is a legal herb in most countries, this is not commonly examined for.

Where can you purchase kratom?

There are a lot of online merchants that sell kratom extracts, dried leaves or both. It is essential to be very careful when it comes to marketing hype and deceitful labels. Always ensure to look for a reputable source. In truth, there have been issues with a few vendors who sell counterfeit kratom and some even debase or alter kratom with other herbs.

When searching for kratom, keep in mind that finding the right place where to purchase this herb is somewhat daunting considering there are countless of websites out there to select from. However, the good news is that a good way to ponder on when picking a kratom vendor is to check their website and observe if they have contact details listed on the contact page. If there is no contact page, you may consider trying another site.

But, if you decide to stick with the website, ensure that they have workable contact form. If you have any queries or concerns, see to it that the vendors' site has complete information and contact the firm if you have queries which the site does not respond to. In case that you do not receive quick response, consider looking for other sites.

Aside from these, another indication of a reputable kratom vendor website is excellent customer service. Also, consider going over the vendor reviews which are found on the web or in forums where users of this product post some reviews of the product such as the quality, customer service and pricing. Likewise, since your orders are being placed via the internet, ensure that the website comes with Secure Sockets Layer or SSL certificate to guarantee that your transaction data is encrypted.

Q AND A

Kratom and drug tests

In general and wherever the consumption is legal, it is not even looked for in drug tests. However, there is an exception to that rule which pertains to athletes. Kratom is a stimulant and a pain killer, therefore it is considered as a substance that can enhance an athlete's performance and falls under the provisions of the prohibited substance list.

In areas where the consumption is illegal, the general drug tests will not detect Kratom. However it is possible to detect the existence of the constituent alkaloids in the bodily fluids with more specialized tests.

Purchasing Kratom

This is where it gets interesting. The general rule of thumb says that if you go online you will find plenty of merchants that sell leaves (fresh or dried), extracts, capsules, powder or all of the above.

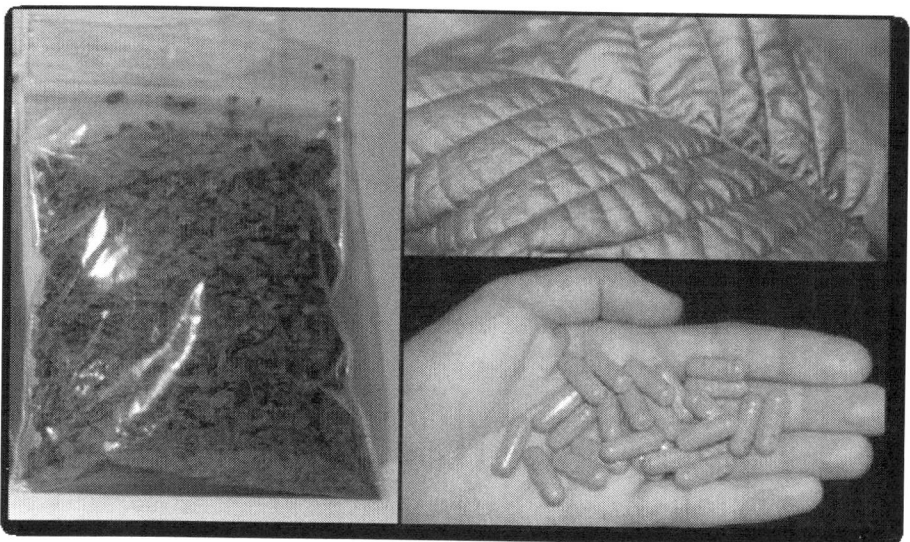

There have been documented cases where the merchants were actually selling other herbs that they have mislabeled as "kratom" or that the substance they were selling was not pure kratom but a mixture called "krypton kratom" which was devised as a means to circumvent the legal provisions in countries that the possession of the herb is illegal.

Both the above practices have resulted in severe problems, even deaths, which added more to the debate against kratom. However, it must be made clear that these cases where not related to the effects of kratom itself but to the effects of whatever other drugs these merchants were selling and to the mixture with other substances.

If you want to purchase kratom online you need to make sure that the seller is a reputable and trustworthy one. It is best if you placed your preference to a local herb store which may not provide all the options for buying but it is more trustworthy as it can be held liable if something happens.

Cultivating the tree

Repeating the warning about the legality of possessing the herb in your jurisdiction, kratom can be cultivated either as a tree or as a potted plant. To successfully do so, here is what you need to know:

a) The environment should be humid and rather warm. Kratom does not grow in cold climates and is not tolerant of frost.
b) As long as the weather is sufficiently warm they can grow outside. In winter months, potted plants must be relocated indoors and provisions made for adequate ventilation especially during the night.
c) During the phase they are actively growing, light fertilization every few weeks is required. After that phase no fertilization is necessary.
d) Cuttings can propagate the plant.
e) Cut back is a necessity for the potted plants as they can easily outgrow their containing vessel given the appropriate environment.

Known legal status

Australia, Burma (officially Myanmar), Denmark, Malaysia and Thailand completely prohibit the use, cultivation and possession of Kratom with penalties that very from 500 dollars to years of incarceration.

In the United States it is legal to possess but it is included in the list of Drugs and Chemicals of Concern, pending the full evaluation from the FDA. On that subject as of Jun 09 2015 there is an import alert which enforces the seizure of certain shipments from a number of vendors.

Indiana is the one and only state that as of 2012 has banned not kratom itself but its content of alkaloid chemicals. The wording of the legislation led to a controversy about the non-synthetic status of kratom itself which, until the issue is resolved, remains legal.

Iowa, Louisiana and Massachusetts have included it in the controlled substances list and imposed an age limit of 18 before it is legal to use, possess and purchase kratom. Taking into account that the Thais themselves do not use it until they are 25, it may make sense if the reason behind this limit was further researched. It could very well be that the chemistry of adolescence may not be conducive to the effects.

It is evident that the legislation bodies are moving towards banning or restricting the use of kratom. To change this situation the International Institute which is the international branch of the Institute of Political Studies has begun a world-wide campaign of informing the general public about the beneficial properties of the plant and that the efforts to legally control it are unfounded and motivated by other interests instead of the possible health hazards.

This is the subject of the next chapter in which will cover the last remaining issues involved.

THE ADVOCACY IN FAVOUR OF KRATOM

The Transnational Institute is based in Amsterdam and its mandate is to challenge the incorrect governmental and corporate policies and suggest courses of action that are unbiased and sustainable. Each time it proposes a solution it attaches an analysis meant to provide the truth and viability of the claim.

In reference to kratom the campaign they have launched is based upon the same premise that the restrictive legislation is. That there is not enough research studies to provide an adequate basis for resolving the issue.

However, instead of choosing to opt for the negative side of the coin, which says that if we do not know enough about something it's best that we restrict or ban it until we do, TNI focuses on a few established realities and the results of a number of independent studies conducted on the matter.

Here is what they base their campaign on:

A) **Decriminalization of kratom is essential to its research**. Since it is the premise of the legislation that without evidence to the contrary, kratom is considered as a risk to public health, TNI has shown that the eradication of the plants at the locations where it grows naturally does not allow for any research from the organizations that the same legislation bodies adhere to, to prove or disprove the evidence to the contrary.

   In legal terms this is the same as not allowing the defendant to prove his or her innocence.

B) **The motives for controlling kratom are political, economic and not health-related.**
Kratom is cheaper than opium. This is why it is completely outlawed in Southeast Asia where the bulk of the income comes from the opiate derivatives which is a multibillion dollar business. Just like Colombia and Mexico are governed by the local drug cartels, the Golden Triangle of Southeast Asia is governed by the triads who have vested interests in maintaining and augmenting the opium cultivation.

While this may be understandable (but not acceptable) for these countries, it is not so for the western countries who choose not to take into account the studies conducted by independent but not state recognized organizations which clearly contradict the disinformation that exists on the subject.

The question becomes even greater when the global realization is that the war against drugs is lost so far and the governments are trying to eradicate the single substance that so far has presented concrete evidence that it can help people get rid of the addiction.

C) **The evidence on the benefits of kratom is mounting.**
For TNI it is an issue of far greater importance than the stimulating or sedating properties of kratom. This issue is the ability it possesses to provide solutions to the dependency problems of drugs and alcohol.

The evidence to this effect is not only provided by independent studies, it is also provided by the limited research that has been conducted by the state acceptable organizations. The results of all the pertinent research are undeniable:

1) Any dependency problems that have been reported have occurred in cases of consumption of more than 150 leaves per day for years and after the user of such quantities has decided to quit abruptly. Occasional and responsible users have not been reported to develop any such problems.

   Even in such cases it is not considered as a dependency or an addiction, it is considered more like a very difficult to break habit. How easy will it be for the citizen of a westerner civilization to find and consume 150 leaves per day for years?

2) Any tolerances that are developed in the body requiring higher doses of kratom to achieve the same results are not of a permanent nature. In all cases that such a report existed, the tolerance was reduced to normal sensitivity after a few weeks.

3) Kratom is undeniably the most effective herbal analgesic in existence after opium without the same side-effects. The zest to destroy kratom clearly has other motives than the health hazards it supposedly exposes the general public to.

4) Even people that are prescribed pain medication that is based on opiates develop an addiction. And that comes under the watchful eye of the attending physician. The situation is a lot worse for people who use opiates without any sort of supervision or control.

   Because kratom acts upon the same receptors as opium, it can be used as a substitute of the opiate based medication after the needed results have been achieved. In all recorded cases, patients that followed such a method have mentioned their ability to end the use of kratom without suffering from any side-effects after their treatment had ended.

For TNI all the above prove beyond any reasonable doubt that the announcements of the FDA that mention that kratom poses a risk that is unnecessary for the public health and that its use can lead to nervousness, aggression, agitation, hallucinations, respiratory depression, tremors, sleeplessness, delusions, constipation, vomiting, skin hyperpigmentation and other severe symptoms, are not founded on any scientific evidence but just on hearsay and disinformation.

For half of the above symptoms there is not even one record to state that kratom was responsible for the effects on its own. And the records that do exist to mention such symptoms almost always refer to a mixture with another substance or to bad product been sold by untrustworthy merchants.

The conclusion of TNI and the other independent studies conducted is that kratom is a beneficial plant which should be decriminalized and released for public use much in the same way as alcohol or tobacco are much more damaging than kratom. Maintaining these in circulation and prohibiting kratom just makes no sense unless, as proven above, there are other motives involved.

HOW KRATOM IS PRODUCED AND IT'S USES?

Can kratom be planted or developed?

Kratom plants can be possibly grown as domestic plants; however, these require to be cut back since they can grow very huge. These are good in humid atmosphere. This herb does not prefer cold weather and at the same time does not tolerate frost. At the time the weather is adequately warm, potted kratom plants can be cultivated outdoors so long as the climate is temperate. Meanwhile, they can be grown indoors for the rest of the time.

Furthermore, in tropical climates, this herb can be cultivated outdoors all year round. It is very pivotal for potted kratom plants to be lightly fertilized at least every few weeks especially when they are still actively developing. Kratom plants can be multiplied through cuttings.

Kinds of Kratom

There are three kinds of kratom and these are the green vein, red vein and white vein. A lot of people assert that the white and green ones are alike, but, in actuality, they have differences. Assuredly, you will notice the clear differences in their leaves because the green vein has green-colored veins while the white vein has beige or white-colored vein. The red vein is considered as the most renowned due to its natural tendency toward superior levels of seven- hydroxymitragynine. This certainly aids in relieving stress and anxiety, sedation and pain-killing effects.

Perhaps, you have observed a lot of names pertaining to the same kinds of kratom that can be really too perplexing. Sadly, several vendors tend to bemuse consumers through rebranding conventional strains with fascinating and alluring new names. What is more, the conventional names for kratom certainly originate from the countries of Thailand,

Malaysia and Indonesia. Literally, the naming conventions compose of Bali, Riau, Borneo and Sumatra etc. the following are the primary kinds of kratom even though there are numerous names available that are pertaining to these strains. Without fail, those names are usually named for the location where the strains of kratom are cultivated and some of these are the following:

- Malay (cultivated in Malaysia)

- Thai (cultivated in Thailand)

- Maeng Da (this is not a region; however, it is regarded as an improved version of Thai)

- Indo (cultivated in Indonesia)

- Bali (this actually pertains to the combination of Borneo and Sumatra. Apparently, Bali named this since it was in Bali where the combination was initially formed.)

- Borneo (This is Indo cultivated in Indonesia)

Please be guided that there are a plethora of names appearing everywhere; but, be reminded that these are still Malay, Indo or Thai or at times combinations of them.

Uses of Kratom

Kratom comes with a plenty of medicinal effects due to its very distinctive alkaloid profile which is perceived as quite unique for a plant.

Some users claim that this herb is an effective stimulant; hence, the natives utilized it as a sexual stimulant which considerably enhances and make their sexual activity even more exciting and pleasurable. In the same way, this drug can also form a mild effect for the brain. All of these effects are felt by the user due to the herb's alkaloid contents like mitragyne.

Ancient people chew, boil as tea and chew kratom leaves. They have utilized the herb for a long period and in point of fact, there are no evidences that reveal someone had experienced some negative effects in consuming kratom at right amount. Likewise, there are no official documents about addiction to this drug; however, they claim that dependence on this drug is probable. Consuming this drug in low dosage is risk-free; however, taking higher dosage regularly or on a daily basis for long period may lead to unpleasant consequences.

Some of the beneficial medicinal effects of kratom include:

- Bolster or promote one's energy
- Relieves pain
- Aid in relieving opiate withdrawal
- Relieve depression
- Transitional substance or opiate maintenance
- Lifting one's mood

Kratom

- Stimulates the immune system
- Comes with anti-anxiety effect (anxiolytic)
- Greatly enhance cognition (nootrophic)
- Anti-inflammatory
- Anti-leukemic
- Lowers blood sugar
- Anti-malarial
- Increases Metabolism
- Sexual Performance Enhancer

Apart from this broad array of medicinal applications and benefits, this herb also comes with very pleasant secondary properties like vitamin content and it is loaded with antioxidants. Not to mention, this made is quite beneficial for overall wellness and other good purposes. Kratom is risk-free in nearly all aspect since there have been no reported fatalities from the consumption of this herb except of course in combination with other toxic drugs, huge amount of alcohol or medications.

The pain-killing effects of kratom are highly emphasized and these are seen as much more efficient as compared to over-the counter drugs particularly when a person suffers from chronic pain or discomfort. Uncountable people have become completely pharmaceutical-free because of this herb's pain-relieving effects. Due to the fact that more and more people are becoming aware of the benefits of this herb, it is expected that kratom will be eventually regarded as a great substitute to opiate medication.

This herb can effectively eliminate pain from such conditions like:

- Multiple Sclerosis
- Chest Pain
- Migraines
- Minor Injuries such as broken bones, scrapes and burns
- Cluster headaches
- Abdominal Pain
- Back Pain
- Neck Pain & Soreness
- Arthritis
- Scoliosis
- Torn Muscles
- Carpal Tunnel

Aside from all these, there are a lot more area wherein using kratom for pain can be relieving and much more effective.

Besides all these, kratom also has its bodybuilding uses. This herb also comes with a little appetite suppression properties and when this herb drug is consumed in the morning, it can significantly aid curb one's appetite for a few hours so that makes it a great help for someone who is trying to shed extra pounds while at the same time bolstering his or her metabolism.

Recreational Use of Kratom

Currently, kratom has become more popular not only in Southeast Asia regions. As a matter of fact, this herb has been sold globally for its narcotic effects and it is commonly sold through internet vendors. This herb provides a relaxing and calming euphoria which is similar with that of opiates and this is made possible by the Mu and Delta opioid receptors. This herb seems to affect the brain just like how common opiates do.

However, this herb has more than twenty-five various alkaloids which come with various effects such as some stimulant properties. Take into consideration that tolerance actually develops and this entails more material to obtain the same effects. It is advised that users do not utilize this herb more than two times per week, to reduce the development of tolerance. For users, please also be guided about cross-tolerance. This conveys that a user can use kratom and create tolerance for both opiates and kratom. Consider the reality that this may cause issue for physicians who prescribe pain medication to a patient after regular use of this herb.

Cancer Prevention and Kratom

There have been reports that kratom can considerably help minimize the possibilities of acquiring some forms of cancer. However, there are no scientific studies to support these claims.

Overall, for the user to experience euphoria and great strength, conventional users of kratom chew 1 up to 3 fresh leaves per day. The veins and stems of kratom are commonly taken out from the leaves prior using and it is also advised to add some salt in order to get rid of constipation. Take note that you only have to swallow the chewed material. You may consider drinking warm team, coffee, and water of palm sugar syrup after using this herb. People who are already addicted or are regular users of this herb usually chew three up to ten times per day.

KRATOM EXTRACT GUIDE

Kratom extracts can definitely serve a great purpose for people suffering from debilitating conditions and chronic pain in which the plain herb won't do. Moreover, there are wide varieties of various forms of extracts that come with differing effects, hinged on both the base plant material utilized and the approach of extraction used to produce them.

a)   Kratom Resin Extracts

As compared to water-based extractions, this herb contains more all-around profile of effects. It is important to consider that these extracts are usually performed through extracting the herb using non-polar solvent and polar solvent; a plain sample of this would be ethanol and water. Just like water extract, the alkaloid soaked polar solvent or non-polar solvent is left to dry and the powder is carefully strained.

Advantages of the Kratom Resin

- Easy storage
- Full-spectrum of effects
- High potency per weight
- Ease of use

Disadvantages of Kratom Resin

- Adverse effects to potency ratio which is comparable to simple leaf
- More high-priced as compared to simple leaf

- Melts in mild heat so this means that it is sensitive to temperature

b) Water-Based Extracts

These are regarded as the most typical variety. Water extract is performed through dissolving a part of alkaloids into water, afterwards the powder has to be strained and then it is required to allow the water to evaporate. This procedure leaves a more alkaloid-concentrated variation of the simple leaf behind. This form of extract is usually pertained as "x" and this means how much simple leaf material was utilized to form the same weight of the resulting extract. Unfortunately, these figures are almost often faulty due to vendor deception.

Advantages of Water-Based Extracts

- Can be utilized in addition to simple leaf to increase effects
- More alkaloid-concentrated as compared to simple leaf
- Capability to dissolve in water
- More stimulating as compared to the simple leaf base material
- Comparably free of adverse effect as compared to full-spectrum and resin extracts

Disadvantages of Water-Based Extracts

- Expensive per potency
- Commonly not quite efficient unless consumed in conjunction with simple leaf

- Can potentiate tolerance

- Not an all-around extract when it comes to effects (this means that it comes with less sedation and pain-relieving effects)

c) Kratom Tinctures

These can differ in their manner of extraction as well as their potency, due to this, purchasing them from a not trusted source can remarkably leave you feeling dismayed. Meanwhile, when these are done well, they can be surely potent.

Advantages of Kratom Tinctures

- Fast acting
- Convenient to store
- Ease of use

Disadvantages of Kratom Tinctures

- Variable potency
- Immediate development of tolerance
- Commonly costly
- Barely provide full-spectrum of effects

d) Enhanced Leaf

This has actually become the best option of numerous extract users because it does not have adverse effects and it comes with high potency. In point of fact, this is utilized by consuming highly potent kratom extract, afterwards this is dissolved in a solution, then the powder or leaves are soaked in the solution and must be allowed to dry. Once this is done properly, this approach can form a highly potent herb. Indeed, one of the most renowned enhanced leaf blends is none other than the Ultra Enhanced Indo or UEI.

Advantages of the Enhanced Leaf:

- It is highly effective for discomfort or other sorts of pain
- Does not have adverse effects per potency
- It has been proven to be very potent especially when done properly
- Commonly well-rounded

Disadvantages of Enhanced Leaf:

- Can cause a few withdrawal symptoms upon sudden stop after prolonged use
- Comparably expensive
- Instant development of tolerance

PREPARATION AND CONSUMPTION

Depending on the jurisdiction you are in, it may be legal to plant a kratom tree on your own. However, it would be required of you to trim it down occasionally so as not to exceed the borders of the space you have allocated for it, or the limits set by the law.

The advantage of planting such a tree is the possibility of having your own fresh leaves which you can chew after removing the central vein. You can also dry them up and crash them into a powder which you can use to make tees or other extracts. The dried leaves can also be chewed but they are rather tough and extremely bitter.

Westerners are more likely to be able to purchase the powdered form of kratom. Some prefer to swallow it as is and then drink some fresh juice right away to fix their taste. The most common way is to mix it with water until the powder is completely dissolved and drink it as quickly as possible before kratom dregs.

Another option is to mix it with some apple or other fruit juice and consume it slowly. Remember to shake the mixture frequently to maintain the dissolution of the powder. This mix has never been attempted with soft drinks containing carbon dioxide and it would be advisable not to try it on your own. Anyway you would not be able to shake a mix containing CO_2. The results would be from hilarious to frustrating.

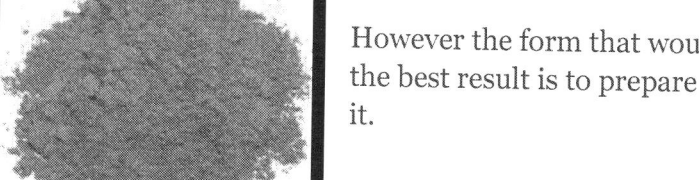

However the form that would produce the best result is to prepare a tea out of it.

How to make kratom tea

Actually this is incorrect as kratom is a variety of coffee and not tea. However it can be produced in a hot drinkable form in exactly the same way as a pot of tea. The recipe is rather simple either for leaves or for powder.

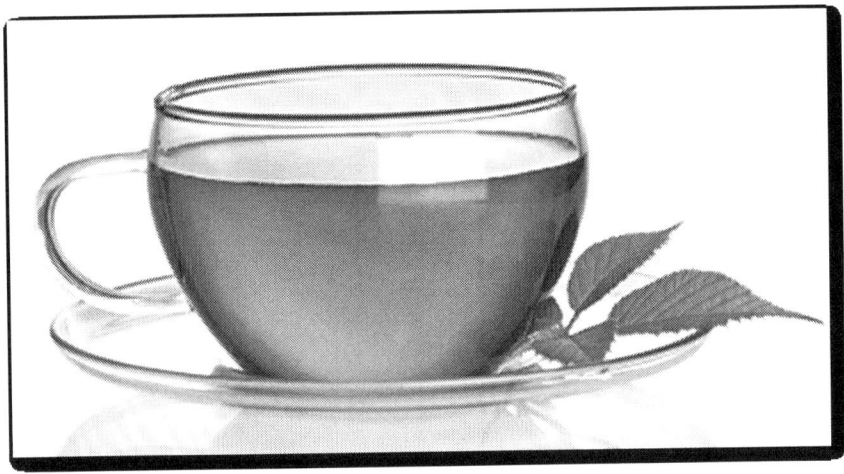

Put a couple of ounces of kratom into a pot with about a litter of water. Bring it to a gentle boiling state and allow 15 minutes. Use a strainer to pour the contents through, in a bowl. Squeeze the leaves to get most of the liquid out.

Re-introduce the leaves into the pot, pour another litter of fresh water and boil again. Repeat the straining process, empty the pot and pour in the liquid from both boiling. Boil until the volume is reduced to about 250 ml. Pour in a cup and drink it fast.

Since kratom is rather bitter, some people prefer to mix it with black or green tea or chase it with some fruit juice. Sugar or honey can also be added to correct the taste.

A little secret here is to not over boil. If the compound looks like syrupy this means that it is on the verge of splattering or burning and at that state it is rather useless.

If you make a large quantity, it can be kept in the refrigerator for about five days. It may be possible to last longer than that, but it is better to play it safe and stick to the five day rule. Adding 10% (no more than that) of alcohol will allow the mixture to remain good for many months (always in the refrigerator). If you can't find pure alcohol, you can use any 80 proof beverages (vodka, rum, etc...) in a ratio of one part spirit, three parts tea. Remember to stir the mixture before the next consumption as there may be sediment at the bottom.

Other ways to consume Kratom

In total there are ten different ways reported. The ones we have not discussed yet pertain to:

1) **Smoking**
   This is a rather impractical method because the amount of dried leaves required to constitute a typical dose is so big that it would take days even to the most devout smoker to start feeling the effects. Furthermore there has been no reference, reports or research that can safely say what happens to the people around the consumer who inhale the smoke.

2) **Mixed in alcohol**
   While alcohol can be a great preserver, mixing it at the time of consumption is not advisable. Actually it is not advisable to mix anything with alcohol.

3) **Mixed in food**

This is more or less a matter of what you will mix it with. The idea is completely experimental and it does pose a few dangers if the chemical contents of the food can react with the alkaloids included in kratom. If you experiment with such a project it is best if you began with very little doses in order to control the effects and should the case be that adverse effects arise, they may be treatable.

4) **In pellets**

These are the extracts we have been talking about. The safest ones are obtained when, after preparing kratom tea, we let the water evaporate. The residue is a paste-like substance which can be stored for later use. This may come in the form of small pellets of the residue swallowed directly or by re-introducing into hot water, dissolving and producing new tea.

Now that we have discussed about the basics, it is time to move a little deeper into the subject, answer a few questions and resolve some misconceptions that exist in the next chapter.

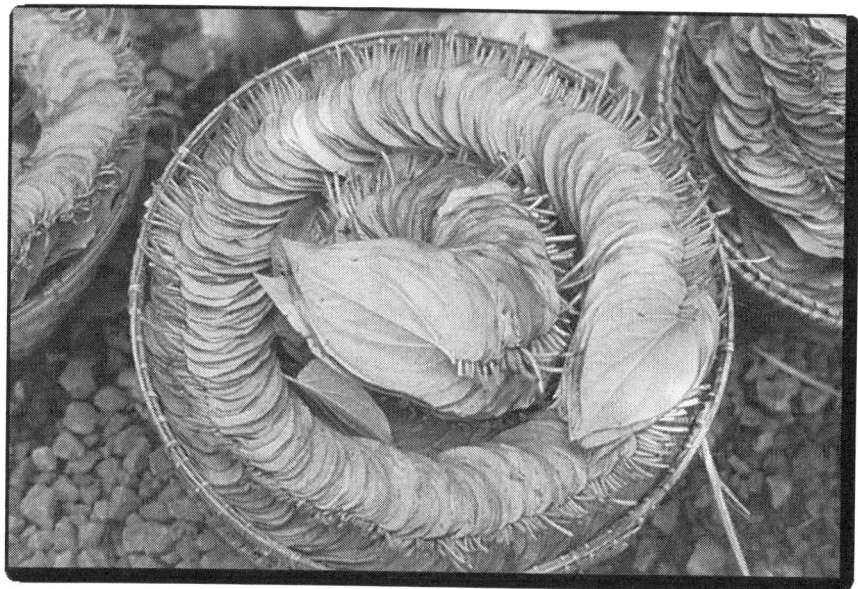

The Kratom Quid

In Southeast Asian cultures, the quid is deemed as the main approach of kratom use particularly in Thailand. The quid approach of use comprises of taking fresh kratom leaves, taking off the veins and stems in one fast motion, roll up the herb and chew it while holding the saliva as well as the chewed herb material in the mouth. Further, the quid works through usually sublingual approaches; however, the swallowed part also has a great effect.

The Toss and Wash Approach

One of the most usual preparation approaches for kratom, if it could be regarded as a preparation at all is none other than the toss and wash approach. This approach is commonly done through:

- Putting liquid or water in the mouth

- Adding preferred kratom dosage to this liquid

- Filling completely and combining the water and kratom mixture inside the moth in order to avoid dry particles get caught in the throat and in the mouth.

- Taking another gulp of liquid (water) while at the same time swallowing the mixture

- Chasing with more liquid in order to swallow any particles

Kratom Tea

This is perceived as another very typical preparation approach, both in east and west. Furthermore, learning how to make this kratom tea is definitely easy and simple:

- Add approximately 3 by up to 10 ounces of water to a pot

- Put the preferred kratom dosage

- For about 15 to 45 minutes, allow to simmer

Optional: strain powder

Tea is regarded as quite efficient since this provides fast onset of effects. But, through straining out the powder, the full-spectrum alkaloid contained in the plain herb may be lost and this can minimize the herb's medicinal properties.

Tea Tips

- Adding liquid to kratom powder and freezing before making the tea can significantly potentiate the amount of alkaloids absorbed

- Putting small amounts of citric acid or lemon juice can greatly optimize the amount of alkaloids absorbed

- You may set aside the strained powder from the tea and this may be reused to assure that there won't be any alkaloids wasted

Kratom Tea Recipes

Since a lot of people are more sensitive to bitter taste, several tea recipes have been developed. Interestingly, one of the most efficient approaches to improve the taste of kratom tea is through mixing it with other mixture or flavoring.

- Speciosa Chai

This approach is quite simple and comprised of a few uncomplicated phases:

- Condense kratom tea to 3 up to 4 ounces

- Add about 4 up to 5 ounces of mixture of Chai tea

- Add some milk, cream of sugar of preferred

The good news is that there are so many different chai mixtures which you can freely experiment with; but, one of the most preferred one is none other than the mixture of Tazo Organic Chai Black Tea.

Simple Flavorings

To get rid of bitter taste, you may add some fruit-based flavorings. It is interesting to note that there are pump flavorings which are available online or at some local coffee shops and these are sold at very affordable costs.

Blends and Mixtures

Another usual approach which has been more currently done by those who do not prefer the toss and wash approach or making tea is to combine kratom. Some of the most typical mixers compose of:

- Chocolate Milk
- Yogurt
- Juice
- Applesauce
- Honey
- Peanut Butter

Besides these, mixing kratom with these flavorings has the additional benefit of letting it to be consumed while reducing the taste; but, with some of these, it may take longer to be digested.

Meanwhile, another creative approach is mixing with peanut butter to create little balls of peanut butter to swallow. Almost any decent-tasting mixture or drink can be efficient. Moreover, tools like blender bottles which are frequently utilized for making protein shakes have been recommended for this procedure.

Kratom Capsules

A general form of preparation for kratom is through capping the powder of kratom rather than consuming it whole, combined or in the form of tea. These have the advantages of being easy and convenient to use.

Some Valuable Considerations

Purchasing capsules can be absolutely costly as compared to powder. Indeed, it is kratom capsules particularly the ones which are sold at gasoline stations and not trusted stores that have had a huge part in giving the herb a spoiled name. When purchasing these capsules, you do not actually know what you're really getting since this is not considered as an approved dietary supplement. This may lead to risks for the legality of kratom and the user. It is because of this why any person who prefers to keep this herb legal must refrain from purchasing kratom capsules. On the other hand, prices differ between countries and hinge on the kind and amount of the product bought.

Products of kratom are commonly supplied as powdered or crushed dried leaves which come in light to dark green color. Beige-brown, greenish or powdery preparations of kratom strengthened with other leaves extracts are also ready for use. Paste-like, stable and dark brown kratom resin can be formed through completely or partially boiling down the liquid from the suspensions of aqueous kratom leaf. Meanwhile, capsules and tinctures that are packed with powdered form of kratom are also sold.

At the time you are prepared to determine your own excellent approach to take or consume kratom, begin by exploring and choosing the appropriate strain for your needs. With aplenty of varieties to pick from, for sure, the excitement truly starts with finding premium quality and fantastic product.

CONTROVERSIES AROUND KRATOM

Founded on the information that is available about kratom, it seems that the actual herb itself is risk-free. Due to the reality that more studies require to be performed, the greatest long-range dangers of consuming this herb are the ones which people are not yet aware of. However, there are also a few which have already been unveiled. Most essentially- and as you may assume from a narcotic that contains heroin-like effects- kratom can also be addictive which implies that people who use this herb regularly will be urged to consume more and more of this drug. Needless to say, this opens the way to the other lasting effects of the drug that composes of delusions, hallucinations, darkening of the skin, confusion and also anorexia.

Aside from all these, the withdrawal symptoms of this drug are identical to heroin withdrawal, with runny nose, aggression, painful muscles, uncontrolled limb movements, mood swings as well as hostility being the most general features. The connection between the drugs conveys that users of heroin will have kratom tolerance and those who are already heavy users of kratom will have heroin tolerance.

Meanwhile, other researchers investigated the deaths of a total of 9 individuals who have been linked with kratom; however, the subjects of the study were also consuming a mixture of substance with a recognized opioid compound which is the O-desmethyltramadol. Be that as it may, as revealed by the research, all of the cases also involved other forms of drugs, and, as a matter of fact, 8 out of 9 of the people had a history of drug abuse. For that reason, it is even more complicated to identify if kratom is really responsible for this; however, this does not disclose that there are at least substantial risks when the herb is combined with some forms of other substance.

Kratom

As with all not carefully researched substances, kratom carries deep-rooted dangers. The greatest one may perhaps be insufficiency of knowledge, but the drug can only be involved in several fatalities prior legislators begin to reexamine its legal status. With that, it is evident that kratom is not precisely another strain of bath salts because the natural drug alone does not seem to have caused any reported overdoses. Indeed, the primary issue here is that the uncontrolled packages bought via internet could contain some additional synthetic chemicals and even though it is authentic kratom, consumers will still be baited into the equivalent of the addiction of heroin.

While it is true that most of reports about deaths and risks of kratom use do not exactly tell whether or not this herb is the real culprit of the cause of illness or death of some people who happened to use it regularly (but because according to investigations, these people are also using other forms of substances which could potentially be the real cause of their death, it couldn't be clearly disclosed if kratom is fatal or risky just like other illegal substances), these cases highlight two pivotal points and these are first, what precisely is Kratom and the reason why there's public debate about its legal status and the second one is if this herb should be controlled or regulated in the same approach as narcotics such as cocaine and heroin?

CONCLUSION

As mentioned, kratom comes with countless of benefits if consumed in right amount and good purposes. Just like other substances out there, once the use of this drug is abused, it can be risky. A lot of its users claim that this herb is capable of giving them some things that are described as wonders of nature. This means that kratom affects their moods and thoughts in a very positive way. It is considered as a very efficient drug to consume when a person wishes to experience, calmer, deeper and meditative-like states particularly when he or she is feeling heavy or disturbed or presently in pain.

Some individuals use kratom because they believe that this drug has the capability to help them feel calm and relaxed, thus, it gives them the opportunity to obtain a more peaceful mind. According to some kratom users, when this herb is consumed, they do not have to worry about anxiety and their negative thoughts are mostly gone. Further, the reason why some users find this substance beneficial is that they can live their life without fears and worries.

In the same way, kratom is described as a fast, effective and strong substance that can be taken specifically when a person needs a strong, quick and effective relief from a painful condition. However, it is advised to consume this herb in right dosage so as to avoid possible risks linked with it when it is abused. While it is not clear if this drug is truly addictive, risky and can be fatal, it is still best to be very cautious and disciplined. Keep in mind that you have to be vigilant and responsible for your own actions.

The reason why kratom is legal to some parts of the world and why it is not allowed in other countries is somewhat confusing. But, for someone who is planning to try and use this herb, make sure to learn more about this substance first, see to it if it is allowed to be used in your country and never ever experiment mixing it with other forms of narcotics so to keep you safe.

For some inexplicable reason, westerners tend to disregard the countless centuries of wisdom and knowledge offered by the ancient people of this earth. The practices of ancient China, Egypt, Greece and the people of Southeast Asia are not taken under consideration at all, if there is no evidence substantiating these practices that comes from scientific laboratories and studies specifically conducted to prove or disprove the theories.

Furthermore, it seems that when there are other political and economic issues that are of much greater amount of money involved than the scientific and observatory evidence, the legislation bodies do everything possible to favor the first ones.

Such seems to be the case with kratom. While the people of Thailand, Malaysia and Indochina have been using it for no one knows how long and can attest to the benefits it provides, on one hand the countries that the plant is indigenous to, seem to want to destroy it completely in order to maintain their income from opium derivatives, and on the other hand the western governments base their laws on disinformation, hearsay and unfounded assumptions of no scientific background.

From all that we have discussed in the previous chapters the issue is rather clear. As long as it is used within reasonable limits and as long as some nominal precautions are kept, it is safe to use kratom and enjoy its beneficial results regardless of whether it's the stimulating effects that we are looking for, or the blessed state between waking and dreaming that leads to the creation of masterpieces of art and intellect (another "small" issue that governments seem to "forget").

There is absolutely no reason that has surfaced so far that says that the pain killing effects have any dangerous effects attached. There is no such reason revealed that can honestly maintain that the ability to help the people with a dependency on opiate products and alcohol presents any kind of danger to the general public.

All the above being said, it does not mean that a person gets permission to consume huge quantities of kratom just like they are not supposed to consume vast quantities of tobacco, alcohol or coffee. No matter how beneficial a substance is, if the limits are exceeded, it stops being beneficial and begins presenting problems of addiction, dependency and adverse side-effects.

Kratom is far less dangerous than alcohol or tobacco. While more research is indeed necessary and urgently required, there is no evidence of carcinogenesis and no evidence of losing one's control if he or she gets drunk just to scratch the tip of the iceberg. All kratom side-effects retreat after a few weeks if a person stops using it and are perfectly treatable. Can that be said for alcohol or tobacco?

Furthermore, the side effects are not directly linked to kratom but more to one's own sensitivities and the possibility of mixture with other substances that can provide a dangerous effect when mixed with the alkaloid content of kratom.

Based on all the above, there is no scientific reason not to consume kratom wherever it is legal. At this point let us repeat the warning not to break the law.

Made in the USA
Middletown, DE
25 May 2017